# The Omega 3 and 6 Mystery Exposed

"Enter the Hidden Powerful World of Omegas"
Are you confused about what the omega 3 and 6 are all about?
Do the words omega 3, DHA, EPA or fatty acids confuse you?
Discover how your body uses these essential fatty acids.

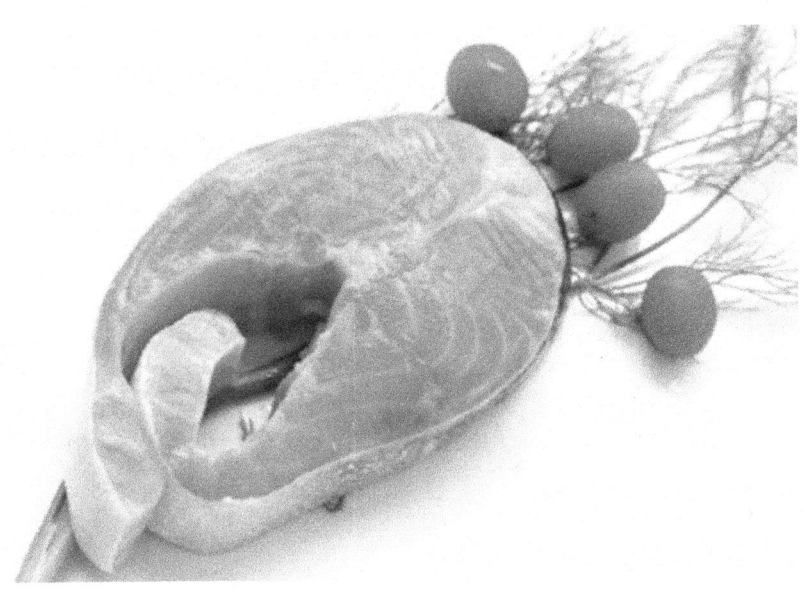

Rudy S Silva, Natural Nutritionist

The Omega 3 and 6 Mystery Exposed © 2013 by Rudy S Silva

Printed in USA

# Table of Contents

# 1: Introduction - What This Omega Book Is All About

**Get** one of my best kindle books *free* by clicking here.

Hi, my name is Rudy Silva and I'm a natural nutritional consultant, who is concerned with the pain and suffering that you experience in your life. I look for natural ways that you can relieve your pain and conditions so that you can minimize the use of drugs.

In addition, I am an educator and I write to explain how your body works so that you get a good understanding of the condition you suffer from.

It is here in this book, you find out why it is critical to know about the omegas or essential fatty acids and how they work in your body.

So many times we choose not to dig into the complexity of how food works in our body. But now, you have the opportunity to get a firm understanding of why you should concentrate a large portion of your health activities in making sure you get plenty of essential fatty acids.

Knowing as much as you can about Omega-3, Omega-6, Fish oil, seal oil, flax seed oil, and various plant oils, puts you in the driver's seat of your health.

I hope you enjoy this book, The Omega-3 and 6 Mystery. **Warning:** If you are on any blood thinning medication, make sure you talk with your doctor about using the Omega oils, since they tend to thin the blood.

# 2: How Omegas Work In Your Body

Essential Fatty Acids are oils composed of omega-3 and omega-6 that you can find, in certain amounts, in all oils that you can purchase in most health food and regular grocery stores. These fatty acids are called essential because you cannot create them in your body, and your cells use them every day.

There is another fatty acid that is call AA or Arachidonic acid, which is not essential, since it can be made from omega-6, linoleic acid.

If you do not eat enough of the essential fatty acids ... guess what... you're going to get sick. What kind of sickness? The list is quite extensive, and it depends on your deficiency.

- Acne
- ADD/ADHD
- Alzheimer's disease
- Arthritis
- Asthma
- Cancer
- Dermatitis
- Diabetes
- Eczema
- Excess water loss through the skin
- Eye diseases
- Growth retardation
- Hair loss
- Heart disease
- High blood pressure
- Immune dysfunction

- Kidney deterioration
- Liver deterioration
- Loss of hair
- Memory loss
- Miscarriage in females and sterility in males
- Psoriasis
- Schizophrenia
- Tissue inflammation

It's a good idea not to be short on these fatty acids, because this list is still complete.

If you are excessively short of these fatty acids or don't eat them, the results are that you will have to deal with various painful diseases or death.

These essential fatty acids provide the fat that exists around your organs, brain, cells, and under your skin. Fatty acids also provide the cells with energy and more oxygen.

Eighty percent of the American people will come down with serious illness because of nutritional deficiencies.

It is not enough to eat essential fatty acid randomly. They need to be eaten in balance. You will need to
balance the Omega-3 with the Omega-6.

Most people eat around 15 tablespoons of Omega-6 to 1 tablespoon of Omega-3. If you are one of these persons, then expect to be harboring or creating one of the diseases listed above.

What are Essential Fatty Acids?

There are four important types of Essential Fatty Acids:

- Alpha Linolenic Acid (ALA) or Omega-3 Oil, a

polyunsaturated oil

- Linoleic Acid (LA) or Omega-6 Oil, a polyunsaturated oil
- Eicosapentaenoic Acid (EPA)
- Docosahexaenoic Acid (DHA)

Omega-3 and omega-6 fatty acids are found in everyday oil that you use for cooking, baking, and eating. One of the problems with these oils is that they have more omega 6 than omega 3. And, it is the omega 3 that you need more of in your diet.

**Flax seed oil** – contains four times more omega-3 than omega-6. It's for this reason that flax seeds and its oil has become very popular. However, as you will see later, your body may not be able to breakdown flax seed oil into EPA and DHA.

**Perilla seed oil** – contains three to four times more omega-3 than omega-6. For this reason, this is an excellent oil to use, but it has not become very popular.

**Hemp oil** – contain the ideal ratio of 4:1, four times more omega-6 to omega-3. Since it is derived from the pot plant, it does not have a good image. But, you can still get in online.

**Pumpkin oil**–contains 3 times more omega-6 than omega-3.

**Walnut oil**-contain ten times more omega-6 than omega-3

**Safflower** – has no omega-3 and 75% of it is oil is omega-6

**Sunflower**–has no omega-3 and 65% of it is oil is omega-6

**Wheat germ oil**–has slight amounts of omega-3 but mostly omega-6

**Olive oil**–little omega-3 and 8% it is oil is omega-6

**Corn oil**–contains mostly omega- 6

You can see that most oils have very little omega-3 that is why you hear a lot about flax seeds and flax seed oil because they have a lot of omega-3.

In recent years a new source of omega-3 was found in the seeds of the Perilla frutescens plant. Perilla oil was found not to cause a digestive upset when used in large quantities. This oil is similar to flax seed oil in content except that it has 19% saturated oil compared to 7% for flax seed oil.

You can get perilla oil in capsule form or liquid online. It's cheaper to buy in liquid form, since one tablespoon contains 7700 mg of omega-3, and one capsule contains 550 mg.

As you use oils, it is best to alternate between oils, using one bottle at a time of flax, perilla, and hemp oil. In this way, you will get the benefits that the different oils have to give you.

When buying your oils, buy them in dark bottles. This prevents oxidation from occurring and assures that you get active and fresh oils that contain strong levels of omegas.

# 3: Best Foods To Eat With Omega 3 and 6

Here are some additional foods that contain omega-3 oil.

- Flax seeds
- Chia seeds
- Pumpkin seeds
- Walnuts
- Dark greens
- Soy products
- Hemp seeds
- Walnuts
- Dark green leaves

Limit your use of soy products. These products use up your body minerals and have been associated various body diseases. The fermented soy products are ok to use. However, recently it has been found that most soy beans are being produced by Genetically Modified Seeds.

Since long-term health effects of genetically modified seeds are not available, it is advisable not to eat these soy products. Laboratory test of these products have been done on rats, which show adverse side effect in second and third generations.

## Omega 9

Omega-9 is not an essential fatty acid, since it can be made in your body. However, you can eat foods, which.

contain it, so your body does not have to produce it.

Omega-9, oleic oil, is a monounsaturated fatty acid and is found in,

- Olive oil
- Pecans
- Cashew
- Filbert
- Macadamia nuts
- Avocados

It is best not to eat too much of omega-9 foods, since they interfere with chemical processes of omega-3 and omega-6.

**Fish Oils**

Fish are also high in EPA and DHA fatty acid oils. Include fish in your diet, by eating them at least once a week. Twice a week is better. Your body breaks down the omega oil into EPA and DHA. But, by eating fish, which have natural EPA and DHA, you by pass the body's process of converting omegas. The fish to eat are,

- Salmon
- Sardines
- Halibut
- Trout
- Albacore tuna
- Mackerel

In her book, The Food Pharmacy, 1988, Jean Carper, discusses the balance of the omegas,

"Now, as far as your cells are concerned, what you eat is what they are. If you eat a lot of fish, your cells are infused with omega- 3's; if you eat a lot of land foods, your cells are awash with omega-6. Critical is a delicate balance. If the omega-6's get the upper hand, as is common in Western land-locked diets, they incite the cells to frenetic activity, spewing out excesses of hyperactive prostaglandins and similar hormones that wreak havoc on the body"

# 4: What Are EPA and DHA?

EPA and DHA are also considered fatty acids. When you eat flax seed oil or any oil that contains fatty acids, your body converts these oils into EPA and DHA.

To do this conversion, your body needs is a little help from an enzymes called,

Delta-6 desaturase and Delta-5 desaturase

It is these enzymes that convert omega-3 and omega-6 into these useful and necessary fatty acids – EPA, DHA, GLA, DGLA. These enzymes also need zinc, magnesium, Vitamin B6, and biotin to help them make the final conversion.

So what are GLA and DGLA?

Gamma-linolenic acid or GLA is an omega-6 fatty acid. But, it needs to be chemically created when your body takes omega 6 and converts it to GLA, using the Delta-5 or 6 desaturase enzyme.

**Now, DGLA stands for Dihomo-gamma-Linolenic Acid.**

As you will see later EPA, DHA, and DGLA will continue to be broken down or changed into other fatty acids that your body will eventually use to protect itself from disease.

A lot of the GLA that is created from omega 6 is converted to the nutrient called DGLA that fights inflammation.

Having enough magnesium, zinc, vitamins C, B3, and B6 in your body will help change GLA to DGLA.

Now, you can buy EPA and DHA as a supplement and save your body the trouble of making them. In fact, this might be a good idea, since your body may not be up to making these important fatty acids.

Why would the body not be converting the Omega-3 or Omega 6 oils to the much-needed DHA and EPA fatty oils? There are quite a few reasons for this. Certain diets and body conditions block your conversion of Omegas into the much-needed DHA and EPA, such as,

- You eat too many refined carbohydrates

- Your aging reduces the power of the desaturase enzyme

- You are exposed to too many toxins in the air, water and food you eat.

- You are overweight
- You create to much stress, anxiety, or fear
- You don't have enough omega-3 oil in your diet (flax seed oil, eating fish)

- You drink caffeine or alcohol
- You eat enough omega-3 oil but you eat more omega- 6 oil (corn, sunflower, canola, safflower oils) than you should.

- You eat too much hydrogenated or partially hydrogenated oils that contain trans-fatty acids.

- You eat too much saturated fat (milk, butter, beef, chicken)

- You eat too much sugar

- You have a viral infection
- You have cancer
- You have diabetes
- You inherited genes that do not produce enough desaturase enzymes or that block the desaturase
- You lack enzyme activity
- You smoke
- You take to many NASID's (aspirin, corticosteriods)
- You use pharmaceutical drugs
- You have eczema caused by allergies
- You have a zinc deficiency
- You eat foods high in cholesterol

You can see that it is not enough to eat more omega-3 and other fatty acids, because having an unhealthy way of eating and living will destroy or block the use of these fatty acids in the body.

Because the omega oils, EPA, and DHA each have certain required chemical activities in the body, it is necessary to get your body to get as much EPA and DHA into your system.

So, it's a good idea to look at the list above and see what foods and lifestyle conditions you have and eliminate them, so that you help your body convert more of the omegas into EPA and DHA.

.So, you should be eating Omega-3 from vegetable oils, certain seeds and nuts, vegetables, and fish. Eat trout, eel, salmon, sardine, tuna, or supplements (cold water fish).

Other sources of omega-6 are,

- Nuts, seeds
- Grains
- Legumes
- Fruits
- Vegetables
- Animal products

# 5: Breakdown Of The Omega Oils In Your Body

Let's follow the path of chemical change of the omega oils and see what function they have in the body and why they are so critical for your health. This gets a little complex, but this information takes the mystery out of the essential fatty acids, the omegas, or what are called good fats.

Let's start with omega-3.

## Omega-3

The Delta-6 desaturase enzymes (that we mentioned above) break down omega-3 first into,

Stearidonic Acid

Then the delta-5 desaturase enzyme breaks down Stearidonic Acid into,

EPA (Eicosapentaenoic acid.)

EPA is then changed into,

DHA (Docosahexaenoic Acid) by the delta-6 desaturase.

## So, omega-3 is changed into EPA and DHA.

Now, EPA and DHA are further broken down into other chemicals or substance. Now, we're getting into those chemicals that work at the cellular level, which are called prostaglandins.

This is how this happens:

EPA creates series 1 prostaglandins (PGE1)

DHA creates series 3 prostaglandins (PGE3)

## Eicosapentaenoic Acid (EPA)

Because EPA is a long chain fatty acid, it is more susceptible to attack from free radicals in the body. So it has a short life cycle. This means that you need to eat
more omega-3 oil or every day take a good EPA supplement to maintain a good supply of omega-3 in the blood.

EPA is important in the body because it creates prostaglandins. In addition EPA and DHA form the structure of cells walls. They are necessary in the function and development of the brain and eyes.

They also are necessary in the proper function of the respiratory, circulatory, immune, and reproductive systems.

When supplementing with EPA and DHA capsules, make sure the product contains both the EPA and DHA. These fatty acids work together in providing
the benefits and activities necessary for good health.

## Docosahexaenoic Acid (DHA)

You can now see that Omega-3 oils can break down into EPA and DHA. This breakdown process, in the body, is slow and complex. In some case, certain people are not able to produce EPA and DHA from omega-3, because they produce defective delta-6 desaturase enzymes.

This creates a real health problem, if you can't create EPA and DHA from the Omega-3 that you eat. But there is a way around this.

So, how do you know if you are not breaking down omega-3 to produce EPA and DHA? There is no easy way to tell except through blood tests and if you have specific illnesses that point to this breakdown deficiency. Just to be on the safe side it is best to supplement your diet with fish oil capsules.

A Pharmaceutical Grade of fish oil is the best, since it is free of contaminates such as,

- Lipid peroxides (Fats that have been oxidized)
- Contaminates from the environment
- Heavy metals, especially mercury
- Other contaminates that get filtered out

Expect to pay more for the Pharmaceutical Grade fish oil. Better yet, it is recommended that you eat fish twice a week and to supplement with fish oil by 2000 – 5000 mg each day taken at meal time.

Make sure you use a fish oil supplement that contains vitamin E to protect the oil from oxidation. Now, let's look at how Omega-6 chemically changes.

## Omega-6

Delta-6 desaturase enzymes and specific Vitamins with zinc breakdown omega-6 first into,

- Gamma-Linolenic Acid (GLA)
- Then this changes into,
- Dihomo-gamma-linolenic acid **(DGLA)**
- Then into,
- Arachidonic Acid (AA)

- And finally AA can change into,

- Docospentaenoic acid (DPA)

## DPA

DPA is not found in fish oils and only in the omegas. It is a highly important fatty acid and is found in high concentrations in the blood. It is found in harp seals, which have a high concentration of Omega-3 and this is the secret of Eskimo health, since they eat a lot of seals.

Both Omega-3 and Omega-6 can chemically change to create some DPA.

DPA is not available in flax seed oil or other plants based oils. Some products such as Gold Omega-3 seal oil give you plenty of DPA.

Where do all of these chemical changes lead to? They lead to more prostaglandins, such as,

Dihomo-gamma-linolenic acid **(DGLA)** creates series 1 prostaglandins (PGE1)
Arachidonic Acid (AA) creates series 2 prostaglandins (PGE2)

# 6: What Are AA And Prostaglandins?

Prostaglandins are chemical like hormones that come from the essential fatty acids, EFA's, which are the omegas, fish oil, and flax seed oil. They help regulate every function in your cells and organs.

This is the reason why Essential Fatty Acids – Omega-3 and Omega-6 – are critical foods to eat.

These prostaglandins do their work quickly in the cells or organs and then are no longer needed. There are many types of prostaglandins each with a specific function to perform. All prostaglandins fall into three groups and as was seen above come from either the omega-3, omega-6 oil, fish oil, or seal oil.

Remember that,

EPA creates series 1 prostaglandins (PGE1)

DHA creates series 3 prostaglandins (PGE3)

DGLA creates series 1 prostaglandins (PGE1)

AA creates series 2 prostaglandins (PGE2)

Let's look at the 3 groups of prostaglandins and see what their functions are. Two of these prostaglandins produce beneficial actions in our body. The other produces detrimental activities.

**Series 1 Prostaglandins (PGE1)**

PGE1 is a good prostaglandin whose activity in cells and organs gives us better health. They are very short-lived and once they complete their mission, they are eliminated through the blood and lungs. This is some of what PGE1's do,

- Activates kidneys to remove excess fluids and sodium from the body
- Helps improve brain activity
- Helps to regulate insulin
- Improves blood circulation
- Improves nerve function
- Improves your immunity
- Prevents cancer cells from spreading
- Prevents the release of AA from our cell membranes
- Promotes a feeling of well being
- Protects against cardiovascular diseases
- Reduces inflammation from skin diseases such as acne, eczema
- Regulates calcium metabolism
- Speeds up metabolism in cells
- Stops the growth of abnormal cells
- Stops blood platelets sticking together

## Series 2 Prostaglandins (PGE2)

The series 2 prostaglandins interfere with good health in your body by countering the activities of Series 1 prostaglandins.

The series 2 are useful in "fight or flight" situation. Here's some of the series 2 activities,

- They activate the kidney to retain sodium, which increases water retention in the body

- They create high blood pressure
- They cause inflammation.
- Cause pain

Recall that AA produces the series 2 prostaglandins. This means that AA and series 2 prostaglandins work against the good activities of the series 1 prostaglandins.

AA is created from omega-6 oils and it also comes from eating too much meat. If you eat too much omega-6 oil, you will have too much AA and series 2 prostaglandins.

The over production of AA and series 2 prostaglandins can be controlled by eating more omega-3.

## Series 3 Prostaglandins

The series 3 prostaglandins prevent blood platelets from having excess stickiness and thus have anti-clotting properties. This anti-clotting property helps diabetics to prevent gangrene and blindness.
The series 3 is created from omega 3 and EPA. The EPA has a powerful ability combined with the series 1 prostaglandin to prevent the series 2 prostaglandins from becoming active. Their power keeps the series 2 prostaglandins trapped in the cell structure.

Keeping a good diet balance of omega-3 and omega-6 is what keeps the series 2 prostaglandins in check. It keeps them to a minimum by trapping them in the cell walls. The result is good your cardiovascular function and for reducing inflammation in your body.

Here's how to encourage the production of good prostaglandins – series 1 and series 3.

Maintain a ratio of two times more omega-6 than omega-3 in your diet. In other words, use 2 parts omega 6 and 1 part omega 3. Now these ratios are not set in stone, and, of course, it is impossible to know what ratio you are eating.

But the way to do it is to make sure you are getting more omega 3 in your diet then you normally get.

Eating too much omega-6 can lead to producing excess series 2 prostaglandins, the bad prostaglandins. Take a multi-vitamin and minerals with your meals to activate or accelerate the omegas to breakdown into, eventually, the prostaglandins.

Reduce the amount of meat, saturated fat, dairy, and eggs you eat to reduce the production of AA, which blocks the activities of the good prostaglandins and produces the bad prostaglandins.

Eat cold water fish at least twice a week to provide EPA and DHA to your diet

Supplement with EPA, DHA, and DPA capsules.

When you have an excess of AA in your cell membranes, AA creates many chemicals, series 2 prostaglandins (PGE2), which are not good for your health. AA is controlled by DHA supplements or by eating omega-3 oil. You can also reduce the amount of AA in your cell walls by eating less saturated fat – meat, eggs, and dairy products

## Arachidonic Acid (AA)

Here are some of the substances that AA creates,

**Prostaglandin series 2** - leads to inflammation, pain, and stimulates mutant cell division

**Leukotrienes** - helps heal injuries, but when you have too much it leads to breast lumps, arthritis, asthma, hay fever, psoriasis, lupus, and is linked to cancer, and creates clotting from platelet stickiness

**Porstacyclin** – relaxes blood vessel walls and reduces platelet stickiness

Foods that have Arachidonic acid in them are,

- Meat
- Eggs
- Milk
- Cheese
- Butter

# 7: Hydrogenated Oils Your Body Hates

Warning: Do not eat foods that contain partially hydrogenated or hydrogenated fats. These fats are found in all kinds of packaged and junk food. Food manufacturers really don't care about your health when they add hydrogenated oils to their foods.

Good clean vegetable oils are hydrogenated to create shortening and margarine. Vegetable oils are partially hydrogenated so they can be added to many foods, since they become a source of cheap fat and increase the shelf life of the food product.

What do hydrogenated oils do? When healthy oils are processed by bubbling hydrogen at temperatures up to 210 C through them, un-natural fatty acids are created that are called trans-fatty acids.

Your body is unable to use these un-natural fatty acids, so the liver see them as toxic waste and proceed to detoxify and eliminate them. Trans-fatty acids are one of the most poisonous wastes that can be inside your body.
Trans-fatty acids, also, can block your body's use of the essential fatty acids.

Hydrogenated oils also have all of their nutrients removed during their processing; this forces removal of vitamins and minerals from your body to help digest the stripped hydrogenated oil.

In his book called, Eat Fat Look Thin – A Safe and Natural Way to Lose Weight Permanently, 2002, Bruce Fife, N.D., talks about the dangers of hydrogenated oils,

"Trans fatty acids affect more than just our cardiovascular health. According to a study reported by Mary Enig, Ph.D., when monkeys were fed trans-fat-containing margarine in their diets, their red blood cells did not bind insulin as well as when they were not fed trans.

This suggests a link with diabetes. Trans fatty acids have been linked with a variety of adverse health effects which include: cancer, ischemic heart disease, multiple sclerosis diverticulitis, diabetes, and other degenerative conditions."

Hydrogenated oils are used by a food processor, because they are cheap fats, which increase the size and shelf life of their product.

Where do you find hydrogenated or partially hydrogenated oils? Here is a partial list.

- 40% of all foods in a grocery store
- 95% of all cookies
- 75% of chips and crackers
- 70% of all cold cereals and cake mixes
- 80% of all frozen breakfast foods and in most microwave popcorn
- in many salted peanuts and other nuts in most candies
- most restaurants that fry foods including donut shops, shortenings, and the list goes on and on

Ok there you have it the information you need to understand and use the essential fatty acid so that you can have the best health possible.

# 8: How Your Body Uses Fatty Acids

Now you know why the essential fatty acids need to be eaten in balance. They provide you with the right kind of health and prevent the formation of deadly diseases. So where and how are they used in the body to prevent diseases?

Fatty acids are used in every cell of the body. They have several characteristics that give them the power to give your body health and a feeling of well-being,

- They attract oxygen
- They absorb sunlight
- They have a negative charge
- They readily reduce lactic acid

**Attract Oxygen**

Fatty acids are needed to transport oxygen from the lungs to the red blood cells that are circulating in the blood. They do this by carrying oxygen through the capillary walls, red blood cell walls and directly to the hemoglobin. The red blood cells then circulate to deliver the oxygen to the cells.

The fatty acids again move the oxygen from the red blood cells through capillary walls, through the lymph liquid, through the cell walls and directly into the cells to where the oxygen is needed.

Fatty acids reside in the cell membranes. Here they hold oxygen so that pathogens cannot get into the cell.
Pathogens cannot live in an oxygen environment, so the oxygen in the cell wall acts as a death barrier. They also reside inside the cell to help form the various structures of the cell.

## They Absorb Sunlight

Fatty acids readily absorb sunlight or light energy. This ability allows these acids to easily attract and absorb oxygen. It makes them chemically active and for this reason they become rancid when exposed to sunlight and oxygen.

This is the reason why you need to keep them in the refrigerator after you open their container. Always buy them in dark containers or dark bottles.

They Have a Negative Charge

With the negative charge that they have, fatty acids are active in many chemical reactions in the body. This negative charge keeps the fatty acid molecules dispersed and prevents them from clumping together.

This ability to keep dispersed, gives the fatty acids the power to move toxic material throughout the body and eventually to the channels of elimination – skin, lungs, colon, kidney, lymphatic system and kidneys.

This flow of electrons through the body helps to recharge the body and to promote brain and nerve functions.

In a more complex reaction, Udo Erasmus, in his book called, Fats and Oils – The complete Guide to Fats and Oils in Health and Nutrition, describes how fatty acid are involved in the movement of energy,

"The negative charge, also, makes the essential fatty acids weakly basic (as opposed to acidic), and able to form weak hydrogen bonds with weak acid groups, such as the sulphydryl groups found in proteins. Sulphydryl groups are especially important in oscillating reactions, which take place between them and the double bonds of the essential fatty acids.

They allow the one-way movement of electrons and energy in molecules to take place. According to one to the world's best chemists, the Nobel Laureate Linus Pauling, such movement is required to make possible the chemical reactions on which life depends."

## Readily Reduce Lactic Acid

Both omega-3 and omega-6 help change lactic acid, which occurs during strenuous work or exercise, into water and carbon dioxide. This is important because without these omegas, the body would have to depend solely on minerals to neutralize these acids.

If too much acid is created in your body, minerals can be depleted and your body can become acidic, which would invite all kinds of parasites and pathogens to set up household in your body.

Essential Fatty Acids provide the chemical activity necessary for proper health in the,

- Brain
- Adrenal gland
- Sex glands
- Liver
- Retina
- Inner ear

As we have seen these fatty acids function inside every cell, in the cell walls, in the blood, and in all organs.

Here is a list of some of the uses and activities that essential fatty acids perform. They,

- Form cell structure throughout the body including organs
- Regulate the cell membrane activity
- Form at least 60% of the brain
- Form the structure of hormones, prostaglandins, and cholesterol
- Have a role in the body's immune system
- Contribute to the proper function for sexual organs
- Provide the oil that is secreted by the sebaceous gland.
- Provide energy for bodily functions
- Provide fat in fat cells before body protein is used for energy in fasts or starvations
- Help reduce the risk of heart diseases
- Provide lubrication to joints
- Improve skin, hair and nail health
- Help reduce the risk of diabetes
- Increase the absorption of vitamins and minerals

# 9: Your Essential Fatty Acid Daily Requirements

Here is the daily omega requirement that most people need to take.

- 3-6 grams of linoleic – omega-6 fatty acid

- 1.5-3 grams of linolenic – omega-3 fatty acid

For treatment of specific diseases, increase amounts of the fatty acids are required. The actual amounts will depend on the type of illness, the health of the individual, and the diet that they eat. A guideline to the amount needed is,

- Linoleic – omega-6........9-30 grams per day

- Linolenic – omega-3......6 grams per day

When eating or taking fatty acid supplements, it is important to also make sure you are eating or supplementing with the following nutrients,
Overall fat in your diet

Normally, the amount of fat that you should have in your diet is 15 – 20% of the overall calories that you eat every day. The breakdown of the types of fats that you should eat is,

- 3-4% saturated fat

- 5-7% omega-6

- 2.5-3.5% omega-3

- 5-10% omega-9
- Vitamin A
- Vitamin C
- Vitamin B3, B6
- Zinc

For children and for yourself, mixing honey and flax seed oil is one way to eat the omega-3 oils.
Digesting fats

Some of you may have problems digesting fatty acids and saturated fats. This may occur because you,
- Don't have sufficient enzymes to digest fats
- Don't have any fat digestive enzymes
- Had your gallbladder removed
- Have a weak pancreas

Whatever the case, you should be supplementing your diet with digestive enzymes. Since most fats are digested in the small intestine, just passed your stomach, you should be taking enteric digestive enzymes.

Enteric enzymes are coated so that they are not used up in the stomach and can reach the small intestine where most of the fats are digested.

Even though you may have problems digesting unsaturated fats, you may be digesting the fatty acids. You can improve the digestion of these fatty acids by mixing them with cottage cheese. When mixing flax seed oil with cottage cheese, the protein in the cottage cheese makes the oil more digestible.
Storing the essential fatty acids

The fatty acids and ground up flax seeds are sensitive to the environment and to how they are processed and packaged.

Improper handling of these oil will cause them to deteriorate and loss their potency.

The essential fatty acids are sensitive to,

- Air
- Heat
- Light

## Air

Oxygen from the air reacts quickly with the fatty acids. This oxidation, of these oils, results in deterioration of the oils causing them to go bad. When using these oils keep the bottles close when they are not in use.

## Heat

Heating the fatty acids causes them to chemically change into molecules that are harmful to your health. This is one reason why you should never use them to cook food or adding to cooking food.

If manufacturers do not take the precautions to package and process these oils in dark or opaque bottles, the heat and light will destroy the value of these oils.

## Light

Light is extremely detrimental to fatty acids. When light hits the fatty acids and oxygen is available, it speeds up the oxidation of these oils by 1000 times. Under these conditions, the oils quickly become rancid.

Light produces free radicals in the oils, which in turn create various chemicals that are harmful to your body. The best conditions for using and storing the essential oils are,

- Buy essential oils in darkened or opaque bottles or containers.
- After opening these oils, store them in the refrigerator
- Use these oils then quickly return them to their dark, heatless, and air free location.

# 10: Fatty Acids For Your Skin Health

The skin is one of the body's elimination channels. This means that the skin activity is used as one method to eliminate waste and toxins from within the body. The skin is expected to help.

- Regulate your body's fluid temperature

- Protect you from the sun's UV light

- Protect you from the outside environment

- Release internal body toxins by sweating

- Provide a surface that makes you look good

**The Skin**

There are two layers in the skin, epidermis and dermis. Epidermis is the outer skin layer. The dermis is beneath the epidermis, and it holds the nerve endings, oil glands, hair follicles and the blood vessels.

**Diet and the Skin**

The best way to keep your skin and all parts of your body healthy is through eating foods your body needs, to work like it should.

There are many doctors, dermatologist, and health care practitioners that say having a good diet does not help to relieve various skin disorders such as acne, psoriasis, eczema, rashes, or boils.

One of the main reasons various skin disorders appear is having a poor diet. A poor diet pours contaminates into your body, which puts hormones, toxins, acid wastes, and bacteria out of balance in the body. It takes a long time for a poor diet to start affecting your skin health and the health of your internal organs, so changing your diet immediately will not give you immediate relief. Changing your diet is the first step in a long process to get your skin and body health back.

Using antibiotics to treat acne further puts your body out of balance, by destroying the good bacteria that live in your body. These good bacteria provide beneficial activity, which gives you better health. Adding a good probiotic to your diet is always a good health practice.

In their book, Healthy Fats for life – Preventing and Treating Common Health Problems with Essential Fatty Acids, 2004, Lornar. Vanderhaeghe, B.Sc. and Karlene Karst, B.Sc., RD, point out some causes of acne,

"To prevent acne and maintain healthy skin, proper nutrition and circulation are vital. Healthy skin depends upon a consistent dietary intake of certain vitamins and minerals as well as the right kinds of fatty acids. Deficiencies in essential fatty acids can cause an overproduction of sebum, resulting in acne. Research has shown that when the Inuit changed to standard North American diets, they developed acne. Far less acne is seen in Inuit eating traditional diets versus the standard North American diet, which is high in bad fat and refined carbohydrates like white rice, pasta, and sugar. Eating too much of the wrong fats has also been shown to cause excess sebum production."

Note: The Inuit live along the coast of Canada and Alaska and are descendants of a prehistoric hunting society that live on bowhead whales, seals and other marine animals.

Yes, there are many reasons – excess hormones, poor skin hygiene, heredity, weak immune system - that contribute to skin disorders, such as acne, but if you have been eating a poor diet, for long time, those reasons can become major reasons for acne.

In their book, New Choices in Natural Healing, written by Prevention Magazine Health Books,1995, the writers point out,

"De-grease your diet, says Michael A. Klaper, M.D., a nutritional medicine specialist in Pompano Beach, Florida, and director of the institute of Nutritional Education and Research. 'Oily hair and skin sometimes are the result of eating too many fats in your diet – things such as doughnuts, and potato chips.

The heavy fats in these foods work their way into the skin oils, contributing to overly oily skin and acne. If it leaves a grease spot on a paper towel, avoid it'

" The damage caused by a poor diet can be seen in your skin, but the damage caused inside your body cannot be seen. The health of your skin is dependent on the health of all other parts of your body."

To have lasting beautiful skin, it will be necessary to change your diet, if you have been following a processed and junk food diet. This change is needed to get the chemicals in your body back in balance and to start removing the causes of your skin disorders and improve other weak organs that contribute to these skin disorders.

In addition, there are other supplements that will be necessary to help you eliminate and relieve your acne or other skin disorders.

In my book, "How to Relieve Acne by Enhancing Your Fighting Power", I have outlined various steps that you can use to help you eliminate or get relief from acne. These steps are also useful in other skin disorders.

Adding fatty acids to your diet will help to speed relief from the eruptions of acne and other skin disorders. In addition fatty acids help,

- Prevent the skin from sunburn

- Reduce wrinkles

- Prevent aging

- Provide skin moisture

- Reduce skin inflammation

- Reduce skin itchiness and dryness

- Reduces skin lesions

It is GLA that will provide you with the benefits that will improve your skin health and provide relief for acne. As a reminder, GLA comes from Omega-6 vegetable and seed oils. Through the enzyme Delta-6 desaturase, the omega-6 breaks down into GLA. It is GLA that will provide you with benefits that will improve your skin health and provide relief for acne.

Since the skin has difficulty converting Omega-6 into GLA, you will be deficient in GLA in the skin area. So the thing you should do is supplement your diet with GLA.

It will also be important to eat different essential fatty acids, since they are necessary for reducing pain and inflammation, improving the health of internal organs, and for preventing fatal diseases.

GLA provides the skin with many benefits such as, forming the structure of the skin cell membrane and keeping the skin lubricated with oil and water to protect it from toxic matter.

## GLA Sources

There are different sources for supplementing with GLA.

- Borage Oil

- Primrose Oil

- Parilla Oil

These three oils are high in GLA with Borage oil being the highest. In addition, they also contain Omega-6 oil.

The important information to know here is,

- GLA can block the activity of male hormones, androgens, which in excess cause an overproduction of sebum oil and leads to acne.

- These hormones are in both males and females.

GLA also provides other acne relief for,

- Skin dryness
- Inflammation
- Pimple oozing
- Itching

**Borage Oil**

Borage oil is a source of GLA.

**How to use it**

Take two 1000 mg of borage oil softgels each day. Take them with meals. If you see or feel any side effects, reduce your dose to one capsule each day.

Borage oil can also be added to your acne cream by breaking

open a softgel capsule and mixing it into the cream. This will provide GLA directly onto your skin where it is needed to control acne and other skin disorders. In most clinical experiments, no side effects have been observed with the use of borage oil.

## Primrose Oil

Primrose oil is another source of GLA.

## How to use it

Take 1000 mg softgel capsule four times a day with a meal or snack.

## Flax Seed and Flax Seed Oil For Acne

As mentioned in the first part of this book, supplementing with Omega-3 and Omega-6 are important diet changes. These are necessary for promoting natural health activities in your body. Without eating the Omega's in a balance way, you will be building diseases that will show up later in life.

## Flax Seeds

Take 1 tablespoon of flax seeds 1- 2 times a day. (One tablespoon of flax seeds is equal to 1.5 grams of plant omega-3 fatty acid.) acid.) These seeds can be taken whole or grinded up in a coffee grinder.

Grind the seeds and use them immediately to get the benefit of fresh seeds and to avoid their oxidation. Your stomach will not dissolve the whole seed, but they will bulk up to provide the fiber you need in your colon. Grind them open and you get the benefits of the oil, fiber, and nutrients that are inside.

You can eat whole flax seeds, but you need to chew them well to break them up. Your stomach will not dissolve whole flax seeds. Chew about a tablespoon in the morning. Then drink 8 oz. of water.

You can grind them up in a grinder and add them to your salads, yogurt, morning cereal, cottage cheese, and smoothies. It is best not to use them in any cooking recipes. Heat destroys the value of the flax oil and makes it toxic. If you want to add them to soups, add them after the soup has cooled down.

Avoid buying ground up flax seeds that you can buy at a health store or on the Internet. You need to use flax seeds in your drinks or food soon after grinding so they don't lose their nutritive value.

Even though Nutri Flax, ground up flax seed is packaged so the flax seeds don't see light or oxygen, what happens when you open the package? These flax seeds are going to be exposed to oxygen and light and as time passes they will become oxidized.

It only takes 10 to 15 minutes in light and oxygen for the grounded up flax seed to become oxidized and lose its nutritive value.

So it would be important to store Nutri Flax in the refrigerator immediately after it is opened and used to minimize its oxidation.

Flax seeds are composed of,

- 41% fat – fifty seven % is omega 3
- 18 % is monounsaturated
- 16% is omega 6
- 9% is saturated.
- 20% is protein

- 7% is moisture

# 11: Improve Your Brain Power and Mental Health

What is your brain made of?

Over 50% of your brain is made of good fat. Twenty percent of this good fat comes from EPA and DHA. Remember EPA and DHA comes from,

- omega-3 fatty acids
- eating fish
- borage oil
- primrose oil
- parilla oil
- NOK oil

I have covered all these oils except NKO Krill Oil. This oil is the new kid on the block. It comes from Antarctic krill, a crustacean found in the Antarctic waters. It provides EPA and DHA like borage oil do, but its chemical structure is phospholipids. Phospholipids are easier for your cells to absorb than borage oil's EPA and DHA, which is in the form of triglycerides.

The essential fatty acids provide the chemical molecules to make Phospholipids. These phospholipids gather together to form a protective barrier around each cell in your body.

If the fatty acids are in phospholipids form, your body can use them quicker and more efficiently. This is what makes NOK oil a more bio-available advanced oil than borage or primrose oil.

Brain conditions caused by insufficient fatty acids are,

- Alzheimer's disease
- Anxiety and body stress
- Heart disease
- Attention deficit disorder
- Attention deficit hyperactivity disorder
- Bipolar disorder
- Chronic fatigue syndrome
- Depression
- Learning disorders
- Memory impairment
- Parkinson's disease
- Schizophrenia

## Making Your Brain Work like It Should

Your brain needs a good daily supply of omega-3. It also uses omega-6 and AA (Arachidonic acid). So this means taking a good dose of NKO oil is a necessary daily routine for keeping your brain from shrinking.

## Alzheimer's disease

Doctors believe that if everyone lived to be over 120 years, they would come down with Alzheimer's disease. It is a disease that once you have it, all you can do, at this time, is to slow its progression using certain drugs and nutrients.

Before you get to the point where your brain has deteriorated to where it contains nodules of toxins, excess oxidation due to free radicals, and weakens and narrowing of the blood vessels, it might be a good idea to start feeding it the food it needs.

DHA is in order for Alzheimer's disease. When DHA is deficient in your diet, you can expect to have memory loss and become depressed as you age.

Lecithin is in order, since it helps to provide choline, a precursor to the memory neurotransmitter acetylcholine. It also provides the chemicals to produce RNA.

Heart disease is closely related to Alzheimer's, because the heart must be strong enough to pump plenty of blood into the brain. In addition, the arteries must open enough to circulate enough blood through the brain and throughout your body.

Even if you don't come down with Alzheimer's or your family history doesn't support it, most of us are in line for dementia. Dementia is also attributed to deterioration of brain cells and support tissue. One of the causes of dementia is a diet that has been deficient in the essential fatty acids.

So here are some diet recommendations,

- Eat better fish, at least once a week and occasionally twice a week

- Eat less fat and particularly saturated fat. A good number for your overall daily fat intake is 15-20% of your overall calories

- Daily use flax seed oil and olive oil for the omega-3 and omega-6 oils

- Take a daily supplement of NKO or Borage oil which supplies EPA and DHA

**Anxiety and body stress**

Stress comes from confrontations or unpleasant interactions we have with relatives or people in public, work, or home. It also comes from the lack of basic needs we have for survival.

When we are young, we handle stress much better because our bodies were born with a psychological defense mechanism that helps you to push down stress and to store it inside our bodies for later release.

The bad part is as you get older your defense mechanism becomes weaker and the anxiety and stress that you have been holding releases and moves into your brain for processing.

The release of this stress and the formation of anxiety come from trigger words or situations that you experience in the now that are similar to past traumatic incidents.

As an older person, you may not be able to deal with this anxiety and you will suffer the pain of excess anxiety, anxiety attacks, or inability to breathe properly.

This anxiety and stress will have a direct or indirect effect on your brain health.

# 12: The Fats Your Heart Needs For Super Health

Your heart has to work long and hard without rest throughout your life. By making your heart work harder than normal, you run the risk of creating a heart attack.

So what you need to do is to provide an environment where your heart doesn't have to over work, and it will provide you with service longer than you need. Take a lesson from the car manufacturers and put your heart into overdrive – a condition where the car's motor rpm is decrease to increase the life of the engine.

Your heart works harder than normal, when arteries and veins contract or get narrower and when kidneys get plug.

**Arteries and veins contract or get narrower**

When you experience emotional upsets, arteries tend to contract. They get narrower as a result of tension, fear, or anxiety that you experience. When this happens, your heart has to work harder to push the same amount of blood through the narrower blood vessels that your body needs. The force against the artery walls from the blood increases, high blood pressure, when your arteries become narrow.

Your brain knows how much blood must be circulated over your entire body to maintain your health. The flow must be maintained no matter what. When less blood flows through your body, as time passes, your health declines also.

Narrow arteries are also formed when you have arteriosclerosis. Cholesterol, fatty substances, fibrin and calcium ions deposit on the artery walls over your lifetime making your arteries narrow. These cholesterol deposits are caused by the action of free radicals along artery walls and other chemical reactions.

Cholesterol

Most doctors use cholesterol as a heart disease risk indicator. Despite this, it is now well known that cholesterol is good for the body. It is bad when there is excess in the blood. Excesses in the body, no matter what they are, always cause problems and requires the body to normalize the condition. Cholesterol is no different.

Cholesterol comes from two main sources:

- Liver produces 75%
- Food we eat provides 25%
- Sugar
- Fats
- Proteins

The liver produces up to 75% of the cholesterol that floats through your body. When food provides more than 25% of the cholesterol in your body, the liver produces less cholesterol. When you eat less cholesterol filled food, the liver compensates for this and produces more.

Cholesterol is used to form your cell's membranes and prevent them from becoming too soft or too hard. A soft membrane does not allow the cell to keep its shape and can fall apart. A hard membrane does not allow liquids and chemicals to pass easily in and out of the cell.

The cell itself produces the cholesterol it needs to keep its membrane with the correct strength and structure. It does this by using the fatty acids that you eat.

Cholesterol is also used to form hormones, such as,

- Androgens – male hormones
- Progesterone – female hormones, men also produce these hormones
- Estrogen – female hormones, men also produce these hormones
- Adrenocorticoid – comes from the adrenal gland
- Aldosterone – comes from the adrenal gland
- Cholesterol moves around in your blood by the lipoproteins called,
    1. VLDL, very low-density lipoproteins
    2. LDL, low-density lipoproteins
    3. IDL, intermediate-density lipoproteins
    4. HDL, high-density lipoproteins

VLDL AND LDL Cholesterol is known as "bad" cholesterol. If an excess of this cholesterol is flowing through your arteries, this excess tends to deposit along your artery walls.

HDL Cholesterol is known as the "good" cholesterol, since it carries cholesterol away from the arteries and into the liver.

In the liver, excess cholesterol is mixed with bile, which is moved into the gallbladder. Also in the liver, cholesterol is converted over to a bile acid. Creating bile acid is one way the liver removes up to 500mg of cholesterol from the body. It is the bile acids, in the bile, that help digest fats and fat soluble vitamin, in the small intestine.

However, when you have a deficiency of minerals in your body, the minerals in the bile are taken out by your body to do work elsewhere. This action will cause cholesterol to precipitate forming gallstones.

## Bile is a complex liquid that consists of,

- alkaline minerals
- bile acids
- toxic matter
- cholesterol
- water
- phospholipids
- bilirubin
- other chemicals that the liver needs to dispose of

When the bile is excreted into the small intestine, the cholesterol is mixed into "chyme", food being digested, and then it moves into the colon. If you have eaten plenty of fiber the cholesterol is held by the fiber and excreted by a bowel movement.

If you have not eaten enough fiber, some cholesterol is re-absorbed by the colon walls, into the blood and passed into the liver.

In the gallbladder, if your body is in need of alkaline minerals, it will pull these minerals from your gallbladder to neutralize body acids, to keep blood pH levels, or to keep lymph liquid pH levels. In doing so, the cholesterol in the bile starts to precipitate causing the formation of gallstone.

# 13: Using Omegas For Reducing Your Joint Pain

Joint pain as experienced in arthritis occurs in both men and women. Osteoarthritis is the most common arthritis. But many people are also affected by other types of arthritis or pain, such as,

- rheumatoid arthritis
- arthritis from lupus
- gout
- psoriatic arthritis
- Reiter's disease
- infective arthritis

As you age, the constant movement of the joints creates wear and tear. Toxic wastes that circulate in the blood, dead cells, and liquid can accumulate in the various joints and cause inflammation and pain. Continual inflammation can cause damage to the joints. In some cases the cartilage that coats the bone ends wears down, and joints then rub bone to bone causing extreme pain.

There are several conditions and lifestyles that contribute to arthritis,

- Obesity
- Diabetes
- Heredity

- Poor nutrition
- Poor digestion
- Lack of water
- Allergies
- Repetitive use of fingers, hands, legs or arms
- Body injuries – sports or accidents

Arthritis is a difficult disease to treat, because there is usually more than one cause. Just working on one cause may not help enough to give pain relief. But, it always helps to know the many things that contribute to arthritis, so that different nutritional and lifestyles changes can be made.

The use of omega-3 is known to provide anti-inflammatory benefits. In the first part of this e-book, the breakdown of omega-3 was shown to eventually produce prostaglandins. It is the prostaglandins that provide the anti-inflammatory results.

So by using the omega-3, GLA, and EPA/DHA supplements, you can get some relief from arthritis, by reducing your inflammation and pain and thereby preventing some damage to your joints.

It is recommended that you use a good dose of,

- Borage oil
- Primrose oil
- NKO oil

Using these oil spread across the day, provides the benefit of feeling reduce joint stiffness and pain in the morning. One additional benefit to using these oils is the coating protection that GLA has in the stomach lining.

The standard treatment for arthritis is the use of NSAIDs and COX-2 inhibitors. These, however, have undesirable side effects, such as attacking the stomach lining. Thousands of deaths and visits to the emergency are associated with over use of NSAIDs.

You can benefit greatly if you use NSAIDs by adding GLA oils to your diet and help to prevent the serious side effects of these NSAIDs.

# 14: Fatty Acids That Improve Your Prostate Health

Most men will need to deal with prostrate disease sometime in their lives. Typically men over 50 are susceptible to enlarged prostate called benign prostate hypertrophy, BPH, prostatitis, prostate inflammation, and other prostate problems.

The prostate is a reproduction organ that is responsible for creating fluid called semen, which is released during ejaculation.

When the prostrate enlarges, it can push against the urethra causing it to restrict the flow of urine. This enlargement is caused by the growth of excess tissue in the prostrate.

The various symptoms that show up when you have BPH are,

- Restricted flow of urine during urination
- Excess urination during night time
- Interrupted urination
- Incomplete urination causing dribbling at the end of urination
- Painful urination
- Uncomfortable ejaculation
- Constipation

**Lower back pain**

About 90% of the men eighty years have BPH. This means at

around 40 years or even sooner you can start to have a slow deterioration of your prostate. As time passes, you will see symptoms related to how you urinate. When this happens in your life will depend on your heredity, physical, and mental health.

DHT and Testosterone Contribute to enlarge prostrate. In the prostate, testosterone is converted to dihyrdrotestosterone, DHT, through the enzyme action of 5 a-reductase. It is DHT that is mostly responsible for enlarge prostate.

## Natural Remedies for BPH

Both pumpkin seeds and saw palmetto herb have been found to be effective as a preventative measure for BPH. Both of these natural remedies have fatty acids and phytosterols. The fatty acids are responsible for blocking the action of 5 a-reductase, which produces DHT.

The saw palmetto has a phytosterol called beta-sitosterol, which is highly active against BPH. You can get beta- sitosterol 1000's of times stronger than what you get in saw palmetto in supplements These super strength capsules is available on the Internet at,

- Low cost beta-sitosterol
- High cost beta-sitosterol complex

The essential fatty acids also provide relief for BPH. The GLA found in borage and evening primrose oil has been found to inhibit the action of 5 a-reductase, which converts testosterone to DHT. Recall that DHT builds extra tissue in the prostate causing it to enlarge.

Using both beta-sitosterols and GLA is an effective means of providing the prostate with the nutrients that can give it health.

# 15: Omegas That Reduce Breast Pain

Breast cancer is a disease that is on the rise. Women dread hearing those words coming from their doctor. To provide an even chance of side stepping this disease, diet has become a critical determining lifestyle. Around 34% of all the causes of cancer are diet-related.

One in Eight women will get breast cancer and 1 in 4 of these women will die. This is the leading cause of death in middle-aged women. So what are some of the causes of breast cancer?

- Genetic
- Environmental conditions
- Diet
- Long use of ERT
- Long use of birth control pills
- Breast implants
- Blood pressure medication
- A diet high in saturated fat which is toxic
- Excess use of cell phone
- Excess use of alcohol
- Excess use of tobacco
- Exposure to environmental carcinogenic chemicals
- Not having enough exercise
- Use of the tricyclic antidepressants (TCA)

## Fats To Eat For Good Health

To have an edge over cancer a good anti-cancer diet is necessary. You have to make changes in the types of fats you eat.

First, you need to know what types of fats are not good for you. These are the ones that promote heart related diseases, overweight, diabetes, and of course cancer. These dangerous fats are,

- Fats found in all types of processed foods (partially hydrogenated oils)

- Fats found in over cooked and well done red meat, hamburger, pork, pork products, ham, bacon (saturated fats)

- Fats found in chicken (saturated fats)

- Fats found in dairy products (milk, cheese)

- Refined fats such as sunflower oil, corn oil, safflower oil, canola oil, cottonseed oil, and the products that are made from them – mayonnaise, salad dressings, margarine

- Processed foods that are made from refined fats, like canola oil popcorn, chips, crackers, and many other foods check the labels

These foods that have saturated fats are more cancer producing when they are cooked at a high temperature, since this produces chemicals that carcinogenic.

What these fats do is activate abnormal cell division, which results in cancer or free radicals that damage cell structure.

We need a small amount of saturated fats, 2-4% of our total calorie intake. Most people are eating 10-20% saturated fat.

## Fats that promote health & body strength

The amount of fat that you need is around 15 – 20% of total calories you eat. These fats should come from good food and the essential fatty acids oils,

- Omega-3, linolenic oil
- Omega-6, linoleic oil And,
- Omega-9, oleic oil

To get a full balance of the fats that you need, you need to eat and supplement with a variety of different oils. Here is the variety to consider,

- Flaxseed oil
- Flaxseeds
- Perilla
- Olive oil
- Pumpkin
- Tuna
- Salmon
- Coconut and coconut oil
- Borage oil
- Evening primrose oil
- NKO frill fish oil

All of these oils have a mix of omega-3, omega-6, and omega-9 oils. A few of these oils don't have any omega-3 oil. Fish will only have EPA and DHA oils. Use a mixture of these oils and you will get the essential fatty acids and the small amount of saturated fats that your body needs.

**The use of GLA for breast pain**

GLA has been found to decrease breast pain. By increasing your intake of GLA, it reduces the amount of saturated fat that exists in your breast, which causes pain.

You can get GLA by taking,

- Fish oil
- Borage oil
- Evening Primrose oil

Recommend dose for prevention is,

- Borage oil – one to two 1000mg capsules with meals
- Evening primrose – two to four 1000mg capsules with meals
- Fish oil - take as recommended on the bottle

Use olive oil and flax seed oil daily. Use 1-2, minimum, tablespoons of olive oil and half that amount of flax seed oil

GLA is such a powerful nutrient that it has been found to kill cancer cells without disturbing the surrounding cells. In their book, Healthy Fats for Life, 2004, 2003 Lorna R. Vanderhaeghe, BSc and Krlene Karst, BSc, RD, refer to GLA as "The New Anti-Cancer Agent"
They go on to say that,

"Regardless of the cause of cancer (diet, genetics, environment, and so on), some form of therapy or treatment is required to kill cancer cells and stop the spread of cancer, ideally without any adverse effect on the normal cells. Scientific research of recent years has shown that GLA from borage and evening primrose oils may be useful in the treatment of breast cancer... a good alternative or addition to treatments for breast, gastric, brain and pancreatic cancers."

One interest note on the use of evening primrose oil as reported by Judy Graham in her booklet called, Evening Primrose Oil, 1989, is that, "An interesting, unexpected and usually welcome effect of evening primrose oil in some women is that it seems to make their breasts bigger. No one knows exactly why.

This was initial reported in 1981 at a symposium on evening primrose oil when several women, quite unsolicited, revealed that they had gone up several bra sizes since first taking evening primrose oil...All the evidence so far has been purely anecdotal..."

# 16: Final Essential Fatty Acid Comments

I hope you can see how critical it is for you to get more omega-3 into your diet. Without it you will definitely suffer the pain of physical and mental illness.

The first thing you need to do is to get more Omega-3 fatty acids into your body. Do this by eating more fish and supplementing with fish oil to get more EPA, DHA, and prostaglandins series1 and 3 working in your body.

Next reduce the amount of red meat and dairy products that you eat. If you drink milk, eliminate it from your diet and move to drinking rice or almond milk. Add eating cottage cheese and essential fatty acids together.

Then, supplement your diet with digestive enzymes so that you don't decrease or deplete the enzymes,

- Delta-6 desaturase
- Delta-5 desaturase

These enzymes chemical change the Omega oils into prostaglandins. Eat them with each meal. Just doing these 3 things will give improved health that will stay with you into your later life.

# 17: Author And Resources

**Get** one of my best kindle books *free* below:

**http://www.natural-remedies-thatwork.com**

Rudy Silva is a natural nutritional consultant educated in the United States in Nutrition and Physics. He is a graduate from San Jose State University in California. He is author of 45 other books on natural remedies. He has authored a newsletter in natural remedies for over 10 years.

## Resource page

Here are some of the other kindle e-books about natural remedies that have been written by this author. You can see the entire list at:

http://tinyurl.com/b2f7wd3

## Acne Remedies
- Best natural acne treatments: Acne facial
- Effective Acne Treatments That Work

## Constipation Remedies
- The Best Constipation Remedies
- Best Constipated Women Natural Cures
- How To Relieve Constipation With Fruits

## Essential Fatty Acids

- Taking The Mystery Out Of Essential Fatty acids
- Amazing Fish Oil Benefits Revealed
- Omega 3 and 6 Mystery Exposed

## Nutrition Remedies

- Updated Version - Secret Diet And Nutrition
- Secret Healthy Fruit Practices Revealed
- Fantastic Alkaline Fruit Benefits Revealed
- Calcium (Discover How To Use Calcium To Avoid Devastating Diseases)
- Magnesium Nutrition Revealed
- Best Nutrition Health Practices
- Potassium Health Secrets Revealed
- Phosphorus, The Best Brain Food
- A Sodium Diet (What You Must Know About Sodium)

## Stomach Remedies
- Acid Reflux: Fast and Easy Cures For Acid Reflux
- Asthma Treatment Cures With Remedies
- How To Do Natural Colon Cleansing
- Gastrointestinal Digestion Secrets Revealed

## Misc Remedies
- Natural Hair Loss Treatment: Women And Men
- Effective Natural Hemorrhoids Treatment
- Iron Deficiency Anemia
- Secrets To Understanding Behavior
- What Is A Hiatus Hernia
- Best Varicose Vein Treatments?
- How To Fix Your Thyroid Problems: Discover Hidden Ideas That Fix Your Thyroid
- Nail Fungus & Health Treatment: Fix Your Fingernail's Health And Look Beautiful
- Gout Diet: New Ideas For Gout Treatments and Gout remedies for Eliminating Uric Acid and giving Gout Relief
- Diarrhea: How To Stop Diarrhea Chronic Or Severe

## Minerals
- Calcium and Magnesium Magic Body Benefits Revealed
- The Magic of Sodium, Calcium and Magnesium

- Create an Alkaline Body with Potassium and Sodium: Eliminate a Potassium Deficiency
- Calcium and Phosphorus Foods: Deficiency or Excesses in These Minerals Cause Bone and Brain Power Loss

## Men's Health
- Best Impotence Health Diet

## Weight loss
- Ten (10) Day Quick Success Weight Loss Program: A new approach to losing weight by changing your eating habits for life
- Discover Secret Anti-Aging Juice & Tonic Recipes: Unique Juices And Tonics That Create Beauty And Youth

To see all of the kindle books written by this author, go to this the Authors Profile Page or this URL: http://tinyurl.com/b2f7wd3

If you need support or want to promote any of his e-books, please contact him at rss41@yahoo.com and expect a reply within 24 hours. He looks forward to hearing from you and is happy to help you understand his material on natural and nutritional health.

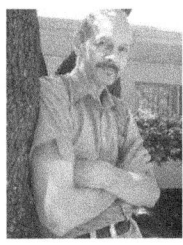

### Give A Review

And, don't for get to give a review for this e-book at Amazon so that others can gain the benefits of what is in this e-book. To you, for losing weight, creating better health and more happiness in your life,

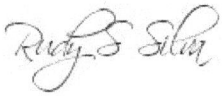

Rudy S Silva